Nourish

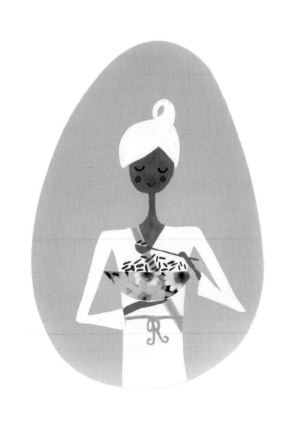

Nourish

100 natural ways to feed your body

Carol Morley & Liz Wilde

Time Warner Books

WARNER BOOKS
An AOL Time Warner Company

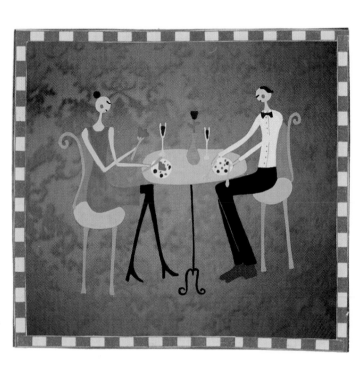

introduction

You are what you eat. Everything you put into your body affects the way you look and feel, both now and in the future. The right food can give you clear skin and glossy hair, high energy levels, a better body, and a happier mind. Add to that a healthier life with less chance of illness (whether that's winter sniffles or something much more serious), and eating well suddenly seems like a very good idea. Today's food may be plentiful, but more doesn't always mean better. In fact, most of us spend our lives trying to eat less, when really what we need to do is improve what we eat. Many modern meals contain less nourishment than ever before, yet more potentially harmful ingredients such as pesticides and antibiotics. This little book tells you how to choose foods that make you look and feel better instantly. And as an extra bonus, the right food is not only nutritious, it tastes great too.

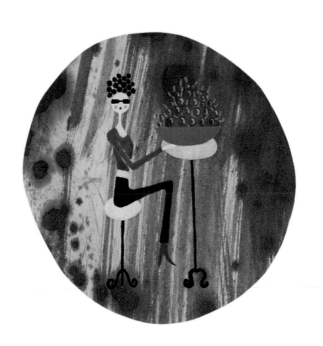

contents

chapter 1 How to eat…8

chapter 2 What to eat?…28

chapter 3 Superfoods…48

chapter 4 Supplements…68

chapter 5 Eating right when eating out…88

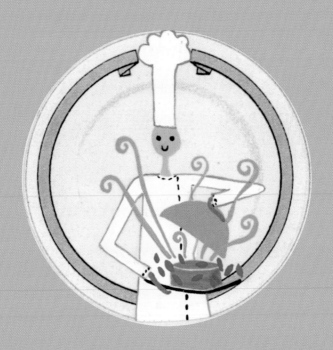

chapter 1

How to eat

1 **Eat too much and you'll finish feeling tired and bloated.** Pigging out distends the stomach and makes your digestive system work overtime, leaving less energy for the rest of you. Eating little (no more than two cupped handfuls) and often will keep your body working well, and stop those hunger pangs for sugary snacks.

2 **Don't delay eating until you're starving or you'll grab anything in sight.** If you've been dreaming of the contents of your refrigrator, all the way home, drink a glass of sugar-free fruit juice mixed with water the minute you get there. That should keep you going (and stop you picking) until your meal is ready and waiting.

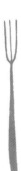

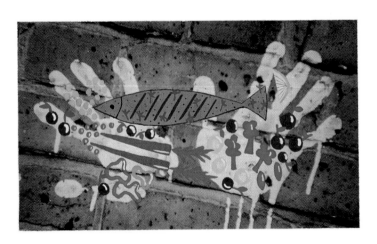

3 When you skip a meal, your body uses adrenaline to compensate for the food it needs. Just a coffee for breakfast gives you an artificial high, but delay lunch too and your blood sugar levels come crashing down. The reason? Your body has no energy left to draw on. Everyone has a different digestive system, which is why some of us stick to three main meals a day while others prefer to eat little and often. But don't go too long without food or you'll upset your stomach by exposing it to digestive acids. Have a wholewheat bagel with your breakfast cappuccino.

4 Can't live without your microwave? Then perhaps you're using it too much. Microwaves are best left for quick-fix foods that cook at low temperatures. Leave main meals to a conventional oven and you can be sure the dish is cooked evenly throughout. It'll taste better too.

5 Microwave rules to stop toxins migrating into your meals:

- *Don't thaw food still in its plastic tray, as the packaging will break down.*
- *Don't use plastic containers to heat up food or let plastic wrap touch food during cooking.*
- *Don't heat food in wax bags.*

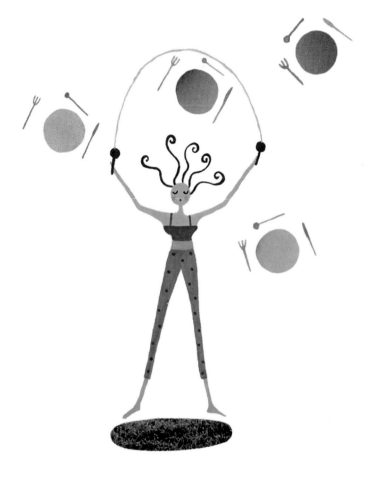

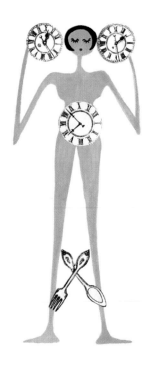

14

6 **Only eat when you're hungry.**
This sounds so obvious, but mealtimes can be more often habit
than hunger. OK, so nutritionists
recommend never skipping breakfast, but if you're too stressed to
even sit still, don't force food
down. Eat only when you're ready.

7 **If you can get into the
breakfast habit, do it.** Research
says people who regularly eat a
high fiber breakfast are healthier
and happier. Surely enough
reason to get out of bed 15
minutes earlier?

8 Don't munch on the move.
Your digestive system needs plenty of oxygen to function well, and if you're rushing around, chances are food won't get digested and fermented. The result? A toxic stomach. Instead, wait until you can sit down, relax, and enjoy your meal.

9 Try to chew each mouthful 30 times. Not only are you avoiding indigestion by mixing food with saliva to break it down, you're also increasing your ability to absorb nutrients properly. Oh, and chewing well helps make you feel more satisfied so you're less likely to reach for something not so nutritious later. Eating slowly also makes you more aware of how full you feel, so you can stop when you've had enough rather than when you're too stuffed to move.

10 Are you sitting comfortably? The way you sit while eating can cause indigestion, so no slumping (and slurping) over your food. Sit up straight to allow your stomach room to expand and get ready for its food.

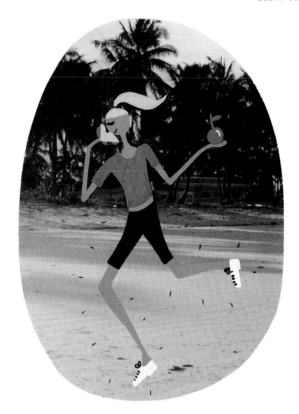

11 **Listen to your body and eat by instinct.** Paying attention to your cravings means your body can choose precisely what food it needs. But this only works for the healthy stuff. Food cravings that leave you feeling low (sugary and fatty foods are the common culprits) could point to an intolerance that may need a nutritionist's help.

12 **Five reasons for you to eat healthy stuff:**

1. You'll get more done (nutritious food is high on energy).

2. You'll look much better (a body full of vitamins and minerals means shiny hair and glowing skin).

3. You'll be in a better mood (no more caffeine jitters or low blood sugar level swings).

4. You'll suffer less illness (a good diet can significantly lower your chance of disease).

5. You'll be protecting the environment (support organic farmers and do your part to banish pesticides from the land).

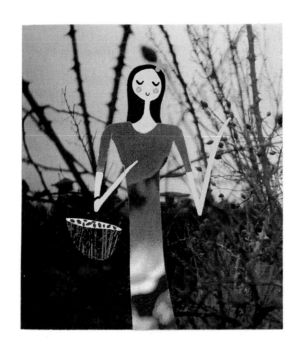

13 Choose good cooking styles that avoid excess fat and help retain vitamins otherwise destroyed by high heat or left behind in cooking water.

Good Cook:

Grilling—adds flavor (and no fat) to foods like vegetables, fish, and chicken.

Baking—again, no fat and lots of trapped nutritional juices.

Stewing—slow cooking that captures the juice for gravy.

Steaming—a better way than boiling to retain vitamins and minerals in vegetables.

Poaching—the small amount of liquid used can be made into a super-nutritious sauce.

Stir Frying—uses only a little oil and cooks quickly to retain goodness.

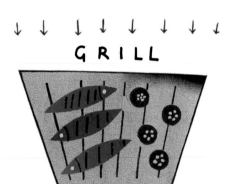

20

Bad Cook:

Frying—fat, fat and more fat.

Roasting—ditto.

Boiling—say goodbye to nutrients in the cooking water.

importance of balance in body and mind. People who follow Ayurvedic ideas maintain that healthy eating requires food that is fresh (the longer it's been uprooted, the less energy it has), grown close to home, and served as close to its natural state as possible.

14 Eastern eating habits have been healthy for many years. Tips we can take include never eating when you're angry or upset, keeping regular mealtimes (which reduces your need to snack), choosing simple meals, and savoring every mouthful. Ayurveda has been practiced in India for over 5,000 years and teaches the

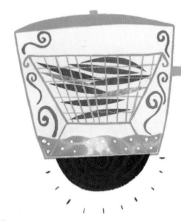

21

15 **Eat at least three hours before you go to bed.** That way your body has time to digest while still upright, leaving it time to concentrate on repairing and rebuilding cells while you sleep. Regularly eating by 8pm will also help you sleep more soundly and get slimmer. It's also not a good idea to fall into bed with an empty stomach, as your body needs to refill nutrient reserves when you're asleep. A bowl of cereal or soup should help refuel you.

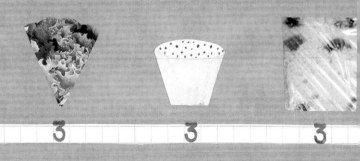

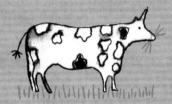

16 **If you notice a rapid dip in energy and concentration between meals,** grab a healthy snack every three to four hours. Known as grazing, a little something between meals will keep your blood sugar levels high and your energy balanced. Fresh fruit is handy for midday munching. But save fruit for eating between meals, as it can get stuck in your system, and ferments if eaten after a meal.

3   3   3

17 Make your kitchen a place you want to be and then you'll be more likely to cook instead of ordering food to go. Give it a coat of paint (but with a calming color like blue or green), clean it well (using non-toxic materials), keep the room well ventilated, and change lightbulbs to full-spectrum lighting (the closest to natural daylight) for a stress-free atmosphere. You may be surprised how inspired you now feel to whip up a gourmet dinner.

18 Once considered safer than wood, plastic cutting boards have been found to hold onto more germs, even after washing, than wood which comes up clean and bacteria-free every time.

19 The days when a healthy meal meant a lump of lentils are long gone. Today, good food can be beautiful, so get creative in your kitchen. Garnish foods with fresh herbs or sprinkle on nuts and seeds. You'll gain extra nutrition too. Plan meals composed of different colors to be sure you're eating a wide variety of goodies, and don't overcook or your colorful dish will turn to mush. Serve food on contrasting colored plates.

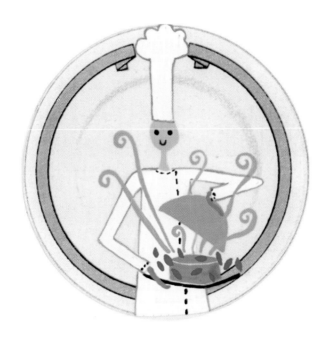

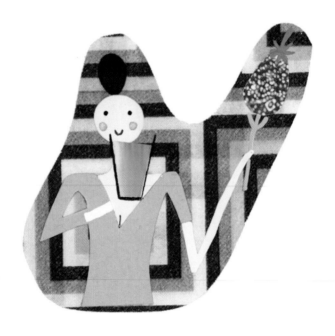

20 **We know you've been told a hundred times to drink at least two liters of water a day,** but don't make up your quota during mealtimes. Drinking too much with meals flushes the food through your body too fast before you've had a chance to absorb all its goodness.

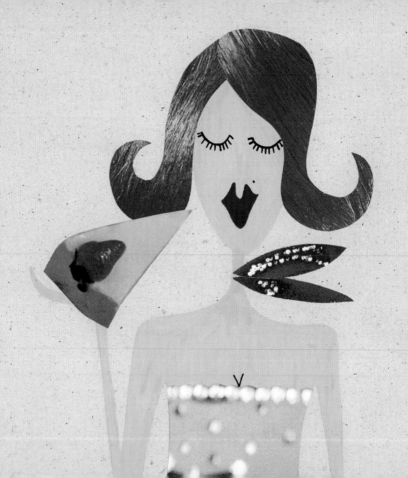

chapter 2

What to eat?

21 Good food makes you thinner. If you eat well, you'll have more energy. And with more energy, you'll rush around and burn more calories. So you can eat more than you ever thought possible and look great. Simple!

22 Food combining was the fashionable way to eat back in the 1980s. Doctors dismissed it, but those who tried it never went back. The basic rule is to never eat protein and starch in the same meal, which means, (among many other of your favorite things), not eating potatoes for Sunday lunch, and only ever eating salad- and vegetable-based sandwiches. The second rule is to eat fruit by itself, and at least 30 minutes apart from any other food. Converts believe the weight simply drops off, but whether this is because you eat less or your body functions better is debatable. We think by merely leaving out the starch part of your usual meals you're bound to lower the calorie count of what's on your plate.

23 Organic food not only tastes better than the conventional stuff, you can also be sure you're not eating a plate of pesticides, antibiotics, and hormones that could harm your health. Cut costs and grow your own. No garden? Then buy a window box.

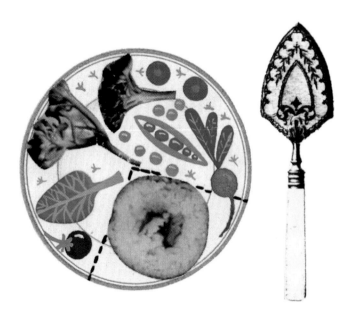

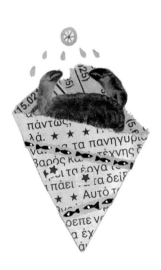

24 **Fill up with fish.** Not only is it low fat, but fish and seafood are swimming in health-enhancing vitamins and minerals. And the fattier the fish, the more Omega-3 essential fatty acid it contains. Why is this a good thing? Omega-3 helps transport oxygen, remove cholesterol, and lower blood pressure. It's also anti-inflammatory and has even been linked with a reduced chance of cancer. Choose caviar (when you have lots of money), anchovies, herring, kippers, mackerel, salmon, sardines, and tuna for the fat that doesn't turn to flab. Just don't deep-fry or you'll turn fish into junk food.

32

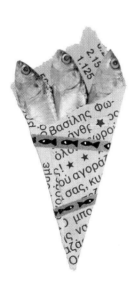

25 **Most protein is high calorie. Right?** Wrong. There are plenty of low-fat proteins around. Chicken and turkey breasts are low in fat and high in protein. Seafood, such as cod, haddock, swordfish, and snapper, ditto. Low-fat cottage cheese is all that and more, as it is also rich in amino acids necessary to build new muscle, and handy, since you can eat it and go. Egg whites are packed with protein, low in calories, and contain no cholesterol or fat, which is why athletes have been fans of them for years. Crack open an egg, remove the yolk and then poach, scramble, or make it into a super-healthy omelet.

26 **Cheese is a high-calcium food and also contains immune-boosting vitamin A.** However, consuming too much cheese that contains a high fat content will result in an increase in the level of cholesterol in the blood; it has been medically proven that this may lead to the development of coronary heart disease. Goat cheese is as rich in calcium as cow's, but easier to digest since the protein and fat molecules are finely divided, and therefore goat cheese is recommended as being more suitable as part of a low-cholesterol diet.

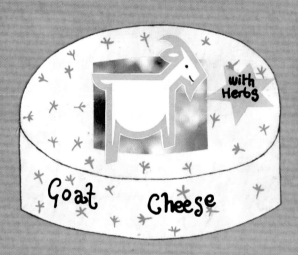

27 **Carbohydrates are broken down by your body and used to make energy.** Choose complex carbohydrates (look for the magic word "whole" on the label) and you can be sure of a turbo charge that lasts and lasts.

Brown rice—a slow burner that keeps you going.

Bread—beware brown bread that looks like whole, as it may just have been colored—check the ingredients before you buy anything.

Oats—a morning bowl of porridge is nutritious, cheap, easy to make, and fills you up for the rest of the day (supermodels swear by it).

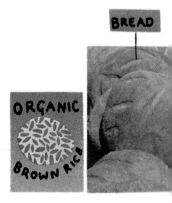

Wheat—sold as flour, choose cracked and whole-wheat varieties.

Cornmeal—buy with added lysine for a better quality protein.

28 **Spice up your life.** Add chili pepper to your food for a healthier mouthful. Capsaicin, which gives chili its heat, aids digestion, helps fight colds, soothes pain, and lowers blood pressure. Not surprisingly, it also warms up your body.

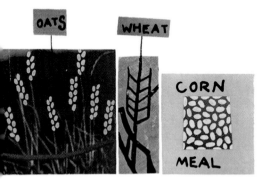

29 **A star of the healthy Mediterranean diet, olives are** high in monounsaturated fats (linked to a lower chance of heart disease). Why buy extra virgin olive oil? Because it's the very first pressing of the olives, without using heat or chemicals, which means all essential nutrients are naturally retained.

30 **Not all fats are the enemy.** There's bad fat (saturated) and good fat (unsaturated) which can help metabolize the bad stuff. As a general rule, if a fat is solid at room temperature (i.e. butter, lard, fat on meat) then you don't need it.

Good Fats:

- *Extra virgin olive oil*
- *Sesame oil*
- *Safflower oil*
- *Avocados*
- *Herring*
- *Mackerel*
- *Salmon*
- *Almonds*
- *Walnuts*
- *Pumpkin seeds*
- *Sunflower seeds.*

Not So Good Fats:

- *Chocolate*
- *Tortilla chips*
- *Potato chips*
- *Butter*
- *Mayonnaise*
- *Sausages*
- *Bacon*
- *Cheese (made with cow's milk)*
- *Creamy sauces*
- *Convenience foods*
- *Pastry*
- *To go foods*
- *Fried food.*

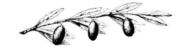

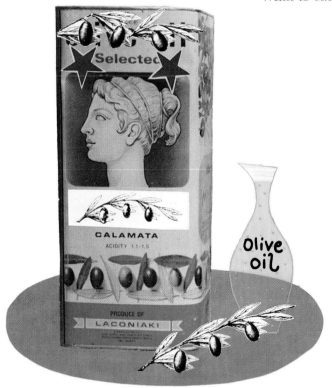

31 For a perfect day:

- *One serving of protein*
- *At least five servings of fruit and vegetables*
- *One serving of carbohydrates*
- *One teaspoon of virgin olive oil*
- *At least one liter of still water.*

What's a serving?
About the size of a clenched fist.

32 Fiber is a complex carbohydrate that your body can't digest. Does this sound bad? Well, it isn't. Because your body can't break it down, fiber stimulates your intestinal walls to help keep other food on the move.

Since it absorbs water, eating fiber will make you feel full without adding calories. Sounds great? Well, only in moderation. Increase your fiber intake too quickly and your body will protest (think unsociable gas and diarrhea). A bowl of cereal is fine, but raise your water intake too or your breakfast will soak up the fluid your body needs to work well.

33 Drinking 2 liters of water a day will hydrate your body and help all the vitamins and minerals you've eaten do their stuff.
A hydrated body will also suffer fewer headaches and have much more energy.

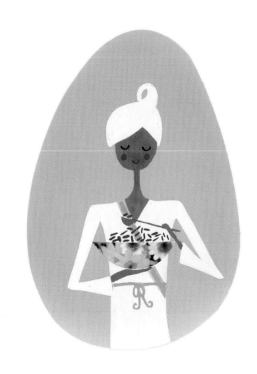

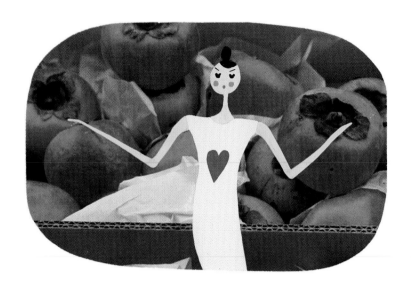

42

34 You can munch as much fruit as you want without worrying about your waistline. For the best health benefits, eat raw and choose from a wide range of colors for different nutrients (yellow/orange fruit contains vitamin A, purple/red fruits are full of flavonoids, which prevent infection). Turned off by your average apple? Then treat yourself to the more exotic stuff when in season (it'll taste better and cost less).

35 Shopping Trolley Stars:

- *Fresh fruit and vegetables*
- *Whole-grains*
- *Live yogurt*
- *Extra virgin olive oil*
- *Fish and shellfish*
- *White meat*
- *Soya milk*
- *Pulses (beans, lentils, etc.)*
- *Seeds (sunflower, sesame, etc.).*

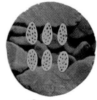

eggs

36 Liquid Assets:

- Still, pure water
- Herbal teas
- Vegetable juice (buy organic or blend your own)
- Fruit juice (buy organic and dilute with water or make your own)
- Red wine (but no more than two small glasses a day).

milk

37 Liquid Liabilities:

- Coffee
- Tea
- Artificially sweetened drinks
- Fizzy drinks (especially if you suffer from bloating)
- Beer
- Spirits.

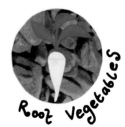

Root Vegetables

38 Minerals make up around 4 percent of your body and enable it to work effectively. Here's where to find them.

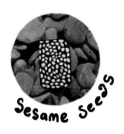

Sesame Seeds

Major Minerals:

- *Calcium and Phosphorus* — broccoli, spinach, turnip, milk, yogurt, tofu
- *Magnesium* — seafood, brown rice, apples, garbanzo beans, nuts and seeds
- *Sodium* — red meat, eggs, fish, table salt, vegetables, milk
- *Potassium* — potatoes, dried fruit, bananas, whole-grain cereal.

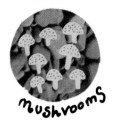

mushrooms

Trace Elements:

- *Iron* — bran, apricots, lentils, liver, pumpkin seeds
- *Zinc* — pulses, root vegetables, chicken, oysters
- *Iodine* — seaweed, fish liver oils, seafood
- *Selenium* — seafood, meat, eggs, liver
- *Copper* — mushrooms, prunes, crabmeat, sesame seeds
- *Manganese* — fruit, vegetables, tea
- *Chromium* — broccoli, black pepper, wheatgerm
- *Molybdenum* — beans, grains, milk, cheese
- *Fluoride* — drinking water, fish, tea.

fruit

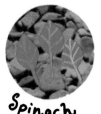

Spinach

39 **It's not the odd snack that tips the scales, but the regular indulgence.** Make healthy eating a way of life and your desire for junk food should lessen. But if you suffer from serious sweet or wheat cravings, it may be your body's way of telling you something. Food intolerance can cause a craving for the very thing that's responsible, so try cutting down and see if your body feels better (typical symptoms of food cravings include bloating, wind, constipation, diarrhea and thrush).

Or visit a nutritionist who can diagnose the problem for you.

40 **White sugar contains nothing but calories,** but substitute it with a spoonful of honey and it's a different story. Honey is an antioxidant (the darker, the better) and also contains vitamins and minerals. A spoonful absorbs quickly, giving you instant energy, and, as it's also known to kill bacteria, honey can soothe an upset stomach and treat infection.

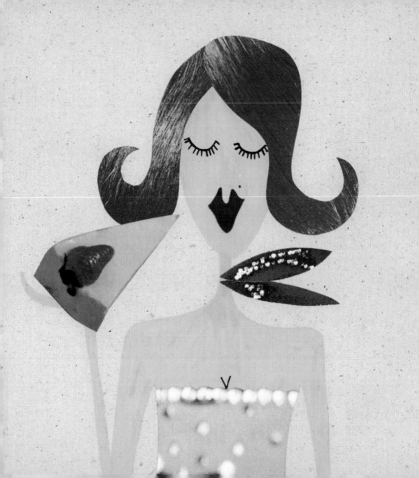

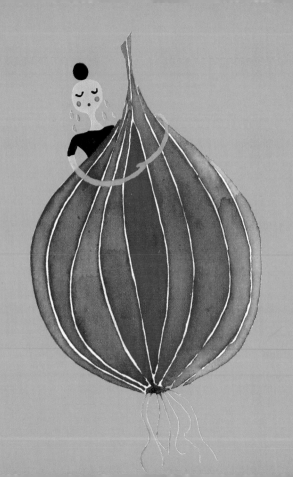

chapter 3

Superfoods

41 Snubbed for their high fat content, nuts are actually super-nutritious and no problem if you eat them in small amounts, especially if they're replacing another high fat snack.

Almonds—reduce bad cholesterol.

Brazils—rich in selenium, which protects against skin cancer.

Pistachios—high in iron, potassium, magnesium, and zinc.

Walnuts—this top nutritional nut reduces bad cholesterol and is high in Omega3.

Peanuts—contain resveratrol, an antioxidant that helps protect from heart disease.

Best to nibble are nuts fresh out of their shells. Avoid roasted nuts, as they have been fried in oil and heavily salted dry roasted nuts contain additional flavorings and preservatives.

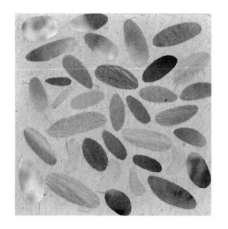

42 Another superfood with a bad rap for fat. There are actually only 190 calories in an average avocado. What's more important is the amount of vitamin A, D, and E, potassium, magnesium, calcium, and folic acid present in one. Avocados are also rich in monounsaturates, which help protect against heart disease. To stop the inside turning brown, sprinkle lemon juice over it.

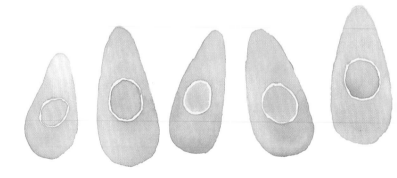

43 **Calorie-free celery contains so much more than water.** Potassium, magnesium, and fiber work as a tonic on your digestive system that reduces water retention. Just four stalks a day can help lower high blood pressure.

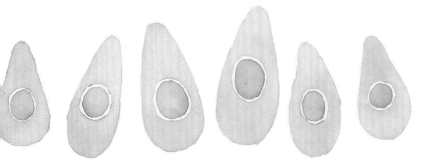

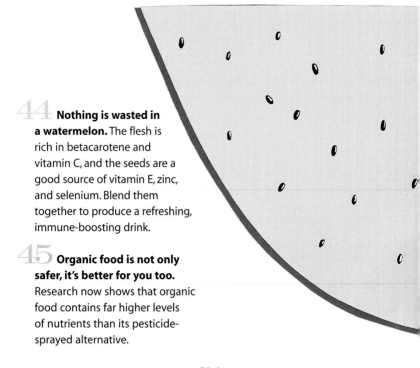

44 Nothing is wasted in a watermelon. The flesh is rich in betacarotene and vitamin C, and the seeds are a good source of vitamin E, zinc, and selenium. Blend them together to produce a refreshing, immune-boosting drink.

45 Organic food is not only safer, it's better for you too. Research now shows that organic food contains far higher levels of nutrients than its pesticide-sprayed alternative.

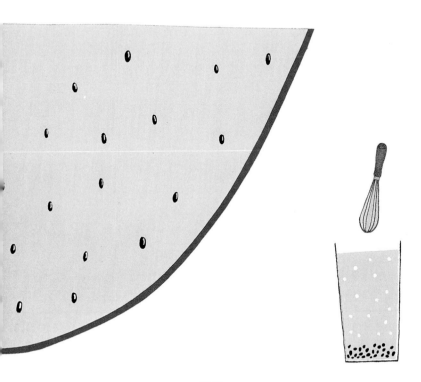

46 **Onions have a long history of medicinal uses** that have been backed up by modern medical science. Not only are they packed with allicin (see garlic), onions also contain a flavonoid called quercetin which helps fight bacterial, and viral infections (including cold sores) and reduces inflammation (beneficial for hayfever). Got a cold? Eating a raw onion will help treat a sore throat and trigger the release of fluids to dilute mucus and get it moving. Cooked onions are good too, but raw is better, and save your tears when slicing by keeping the root end intact.

47 **The humble tomato is stuffed with goodies,** including vitamin C, betacarotene, potassium, and lycopene, a powerful antioxidant that also helps protect from breast cancer. Eating enough of the red stuff is great for digestion, helps lower blood pressure, and even slows aging. Cooking tomatoes increases their benefits, making Spaghetti Marinara a very healthy meal. Research recommends eating ten portions of tomatoes a week (a portion equals one medium-sized tomato). Have a regular supply in your refrigerator to add color to your cooking.

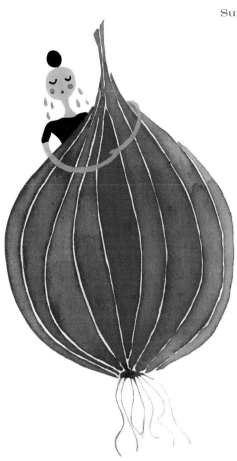

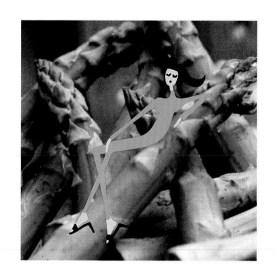

58

48 **It may be one of the more expensive vegetables, but asparagus is worth every penny.** Rich in betacarotene, B complex, vitamin C, and potassium, a spear or two can treat insomnia, soothe cystitis, relieve indigestion, and beat water retention and constipation. Cook in a little water with the spears pointing skyward. Try to avoid dipping them in butter!

49 **Eat your greens.** Vegetables like broccoli, cabbage, cauliflower, and Brussels sprouts can reduce your risk of cancer, heart disease, and strokes. These super-veggies also give your liver a helping hand and can prevent anemia with their high levels of iron. They are best eaten raw (i.e. juiced) or lightly steamed in order to activate their cancer protective properties.

50 **Choose berries with a blue/purple color** (black grapes, blackcurrants, cranberries, blueberries, and so on) and you're eating vitamin C plus a powerful flavonoid called anthocyanidins. Super-healing, a handful of fresh fruit a day can boost immunity, soothe menstrual cramps, help prevent varicose veins, and balance hormones. Studies also show these berries are good for your skin, as they promote healthy collagen, which keep wrinkles at bay.

51 **Apples may not be the most exotic fruit, but their health benefits are huge.** Containing betacarotene, B-complex, potassium, and pectin, they aid digestion of fatty foods and encourage elimination. Have an apple a day after an over-indulgent week to clean out your body.

52 **Trouble nodding off?** Then eat a banana before bedtime, as bananas increase levels of soothing serotonin which helps promote sleep.

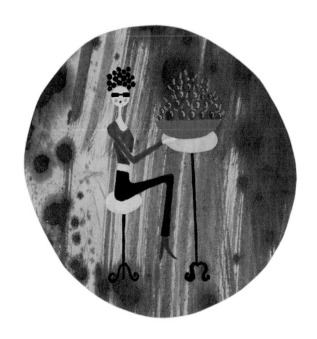

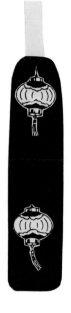

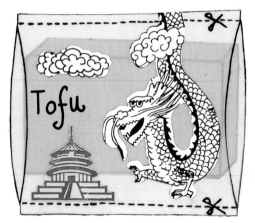

53 **Popular in the East, we in the West have now woken up to the health benefits of soya beans.** Low in fat, but high in protein, iron, potassium, calcium, and healthy unsaturated fats, fresh organic soya can help balance hormones and reduce premenstrual stress, improve digestion, and lower your risk of heart disease. You can find these beans in soya milk, miso soup, and bean curd.

54 **A garlic clove a day really can keep the doctor away.** Garlic is a potent immune booster and contains both antibacterial and anitviral properties. The magic ingredient in it is allicin, which lowers cholesterol, helps prevent heart disease and strokes, and fights off infection. Activate the allicin by crushing a clove with the flat side of your knife, then let it stand for 15 minutes before cooking (baking whole garlic cloves will lock in their healing properties).

55 **It may taste terrible, but salty sea water is actually packed with nutrients,** including calcium, magnesium, iron, sodium, potassium, and iodine. This makes plants that grow in such water like seaweed, seriously good sources of minerals. Proven to promote good health, a Japanese meal of miso soup and seaweed salad will heal what ails you when you are feeling low.

56 **The humble pea is packed with nutrients,** including vitamins A and C, folic acid, iron, zinc, and magnesium. These add up to making a powerful protector against heart disease. Eat either fresh or frozen, as processing won't affect their healing properties.

57 **Flavonoids are designed to protect a plant from fungal attack and bacteria,** so you can imagine how protective they are to the human body. Of their many star qualities, flavonoids help reduce inflammation and thus guard against allergies and viruses, fight aging free radicals, protect against heart disease, and balance wayward hormones. Find them in the pulp of fruit and vegetables (so eat them whole) especially onions, apples, and tomatoes (the cherry type have 30 times the amount of your average tomato). Flavonoid-rich drinks include green and black tea, dark beer, and red wine. Cheers!

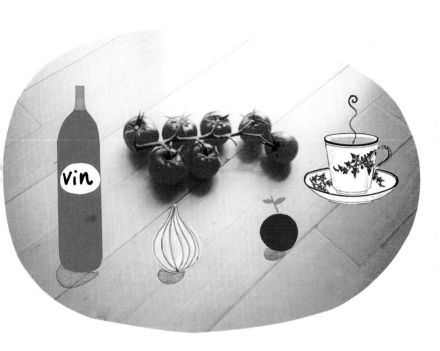

58 Looking for something nutritious to spread on your toast? Yeast extract is low in fat and high in protein, so perfect for vegetarians trying to make up their quota. Add to that a ton of extras like calcium, iron, the B vitamins, and folic acid, and marmalade doesn't get a look in.

59 Buy your yogurt plain, as fruit-on-the-bottom flavoring kills off the friendly bacteria that make yogurt so healing. Look for mind-boggling words in the ingredients list like *Lactobacillus bulgaricus* and *Streptococcus thermaphilus* (or check that it says "live cultures") which boost immunity, fight colds, and help reduce symptoms of hay fever. Plain stuff too boring? Then throw in your own fresh fruit.

60 Taking antibiotics can kill off the good bacteria in your stomach, causing digestive problems and yeast infections like thrush. Fight back by eating yogurt containing *Lactobacillus acidophilus* and *Bifidobacteria*, which will counteract the attack. Eating a small pot two of yogurt hours after you've popped a pill will do the job.

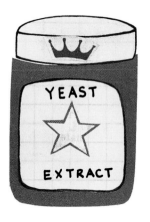

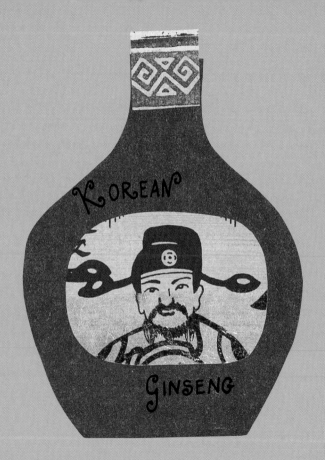

chapter 4

Supplements

61 Lead a stressful life, smoke, drink, or live in a polluted environment, and you're depleting your natural nutritional stores. No supplement is a substitute for a well-balanced diet, but with modern farming techniques making our food less nutritious, plus regular microwave meals, popping the odd pill starts to make sense. The right supplement can help you prevent illness, or recover faster from the one you've had. If a pill's doing you good, you should feel a noticeable improvement by the end of your first month's supply.

62 Feel like you're about to come down with something? Reach for echinacea, the immune-boosting wonder supplement. Best taken either as capsules of the powdered herb or drops of a concentrated extract, fans swear by it to ward off the first signs of a cold or flu.

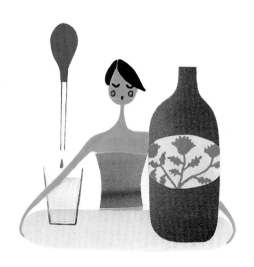

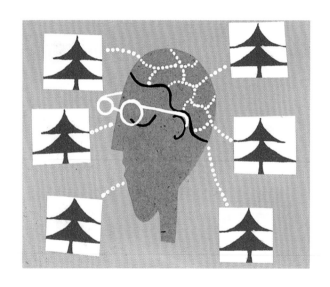

63 The leaf of the ginkgo biloba tree has been used for centuries to treat everything from memory loss to chilblains. The benefits of this antioxidant include improved blood flow to boost circulation, better digestion, and a less hideous hangover. Some believe ginkgo biloba also increases the flow of oxygen to the brain to enhance mental performance.

64 Milk Thistle is a Mediterranean plant that has long been used for its medicinal properties, but is now recognized as a remedy for an overworked liver. Too much alcohol the night before? A couple of capsules will help your liver protect itself.

65 The artichoke is another member of the daisy family that can save you the morning after the night before. A couple of capsules help you feel human again by protecting and enhancing the liver's function.

66 Ginger has been used for more than 1,500 years as nature's remedy for nausea. Studies show it also works well for morning sickness by neutralizing excess stomach acid. Powdered ginger may also prevent sea sickness. Ginger's hot properties also help warm you in winter and kickstart a sluggish circulation. Taking some before wrapping yourself in warm clothes will help your body sweat out a cold.

67 **Chinese and Korean Ginseng have been taken for years to heighten sexual response, extend life, boost brain power, and raise energy levels.** Nowadays, it is most popular for times of stress to soothe the mind and fight off tiredness. Studies show this supplement really does sharpen the mind, improve concentration, shorten reaction time, and give you a shot of energy. Take one capsule a day or sip a herbal tea when you're in need of a tonic.

68 **Take your supplement according to the instructions on the bottle,** as too high a dose could be dangerous. As a rule, pop your pill with your first meal of the day–every day, if you want it to work.

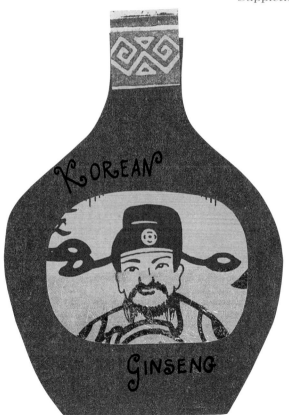

69 Bee pollen is a natural antibiotic and works wonders as a general tonic when you need a lift. The gritty powder tastes good sprinkled over fruit and yogurt. Buy the best, as cheaper supplies can be contaminated, but avoid it if you're pollen-sensitive or allergic to bee stings.

70 Healing herbs:

Parsley—High in vitamin C, beta-carotene, iron, and magnesium, parsley relieves indigestion, boosts the immune system, helps heal gum disease, and freshens the breath.

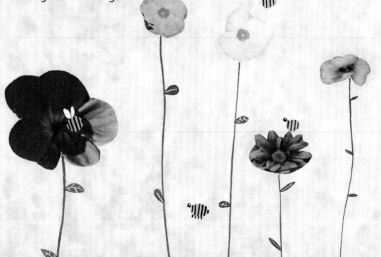

Thyme—Aids digestion and soothes an upset stomach. Thyme also fights infection and can be used as a mouthwash.

Mint—Famous as an after-dinner digestion aid and great for deflating a bloated stomach, mint also works on cold symptoms, including coughs, sore throats, fever, and headaches.

Rosemary—A stress soother that also relieves headaches, aids digestion, and boosts circulation.

Basil—A multi-talented herb, basil helps alleviate depression, fight infection, clear the mind, and calm nerves.

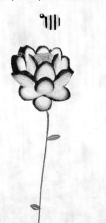
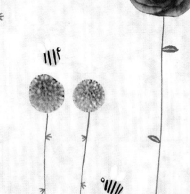

71 In ancient times, healers relied on herbs and spices to treat the sick. Make sure these remedies are stored in your spice rack.

Cinnamon: An antibacterial bark that can inhibit the growth of some common bacteria that fight infection. Take it to aid digestion, control diarrhea (including holiday tum), fight food poisoning, ease menstrual cramps, and counter a yeast infection.

Turmeric: A brightly colored spice that reduces inflammation, making it beneficial for muscular injury, arthritis, and even hay fever. Its active component, curcumin, is thought to be as effective as common anti-inflammatory drugs.

Cardamom: An Asian spice that aids digestion and reduces gas and stomach spasms.

72 Buy the most expensive supplement you can afford, as superior brands tend to be better formulated, which means they're easily absorbed into your body and work faster. After opening, throw away the ball of cotton wool on the top, as this can attract moisture and damage the bottle's contents.

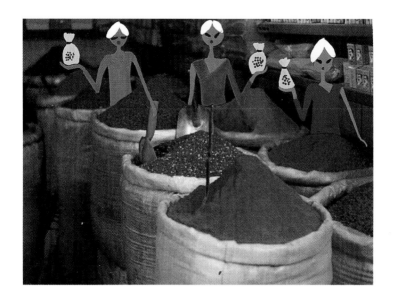

73 **Taken from a rainforest plant, cat's claw is another potent antioxidant that fights off winter colds and flu.** Feeling sniffly? Sip four cups of cat's claw tea a day or take as a supplement.

74 **Wheatgrass juice contains nutritious enzymes and vitamins that can help if you want to lose weight.** Don't worry if you feel a little strange after drinking it. It's just the juice doing its job.

75 **Healing doesn't only come in tablet form.** Here are some herbal teas that can help:

Ginseng—wakes you up and gets you buzzing

St. John's Wort—cheers you up and soothes your aching body

Ginger—warms you up and gives you a caffeine-free jolt of energy

Peppermint—helps your body digest a big meal

Camomile—soothes you to. When possible, brew loose leaves, as they're more potent than the your average herbal tea bag.

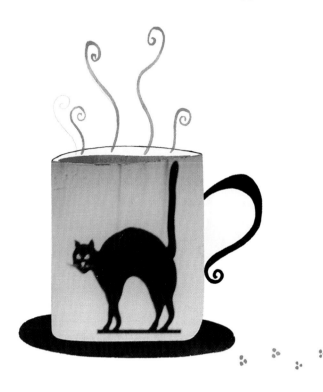

76 Not all mushrooms are created equal. Forget boring button ones: choose shiitake and maitake mushrooms for their immune-boosting properties. Shiitake mushrooms are anti-viral, while maitake ones lower blood pressure. Cooking them makes them more nutritious. Buy mushroom powder from a health food store and ingest three times a day.

77 Antioxidants are vital vitamins for fighting free radicals (a molecule that damages cells and causes aging), and Co-enzyme Q10 is believed to be the best of the bunch. Find Co-enzyme Q10 in nuts (walnuts, pistachios, and peanuts), fish and sesame seeds, or take a CoQ10 supplement once a day to ward off wrinkles.

78 Taken to cure lameness in the 18th century, cod liver oil is known for easing the pain of arthritis. It is one of the few natural sources of fat-soluble vitamins A and D, and is also packed with Omega-3 (the good oil found in fish). Apart from its body benefits (think lower choles-terol and blood pressure levels), studies say taking Omega-3 in the form of pure cod liver oil can reduce severe depression and aggression due to stress. And you'll love the shiny hair, glowing skin, and strong nails you, get after a month on these pills too.

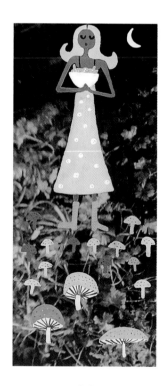

83

Apple
Cider

Vinegar

79 Sprinkle apple cider vinegar over your food for an extra health hit. Containing small amounts of potassium and calcium, this spicy vinegar aids digestion, helps regulate your metabolism, and inhibits intestinal infections. And it tastes good too.

80 **Aloe vera is one of nature's beauty aids.** Smeared over your skin, in slippery gel form, it soothes sunburn, helps heal scarring, and takes the sting out of bites. Drink aloe vera juice and it works as a natural cleanser for a clogged-up body, enhancing digestion, soothing Irritable Bowel Syndrome, and reducing pollution in the intestines. Buy a flavored bottle of the juice, which can taste much nicer than the straight stuff.

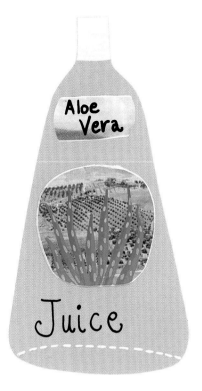

Aloe
Vera

Juice

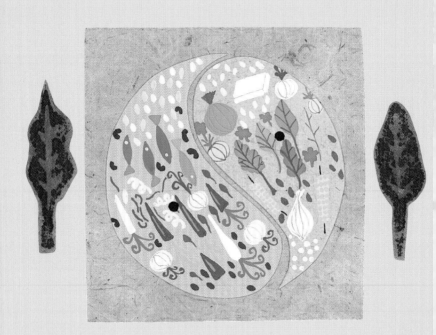

chapter 5

Eating right
when eating out

81 Healthy eating doesn't mean being stuck at home for the rest of your life. Here are some basic rules to make a restaurant meal much more nutritious (and guilt-free).

- *Start with a low-calorie, low-fat starter such as soup, salad, or shellfish and you will be able to eat more food later on.*
- *Instead of a main course, order several starters, with extra bread to beef them up.*
- *Choose foods as close to their natural state as possible, i.e. a baked potato rather than french fries.*
- *Most restaurants offer a low-fat dressing for your salad. Switch and save serious calories.*
- *A heavy meal may leave your body aching for something sweet, but instead of downing the whole dessert yourself, share one portion with a friend. You'll get your sugar fix without the guilt trip.*

82 If the meal you thought sounded healthy turns out to be anything but, do a bit of do-it-yourself pruning. Use your knife to cut off excess fat, your fork to lift away fried, or crisp skin, and your spoon to ladle off rich sauces.

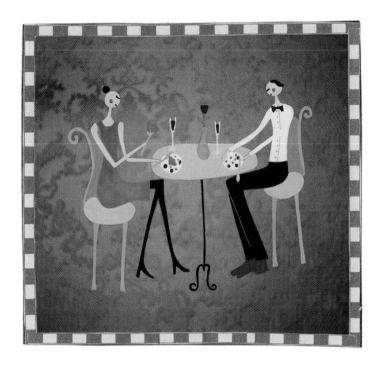

83 Too much salt isn't smart, as it stops your kidneys from filtering fluid, which causes water retention (not to mention cellulite and puffy eyes). Think food tastes bland without it? That's what other flavorings are put on your table for. Make friends with the pepper grinder. Add a spoonful of horseradish sauce or mustard. Sprinkle on a few dried chilies. Trust us. Your meal won't taste mediocre anymore.

84 Alcohol causes a dip in blood sugar levels, which is why, after a few party drinks, you find yourself heading straight for the buffet. Not a good move when most traditional party fare includes (depending on the elegance of your party) creamy canapés, mini sausages, cheese sticks, and salty potato chips and nuts. The safest way to snack is to choose foods with a strong flavor that make your taste buds feel satisfied. That means unsalted nuts and olives, or crunchy Mexican tortillas, and Chinese rice crackers.

85 The best natural hangover cure is a fresh juice to rebalance your body. Beetroot helps cleanse your kidneys, and citrus juices are rich in vitamin C and natural sugars which compensate for the dip in your own.

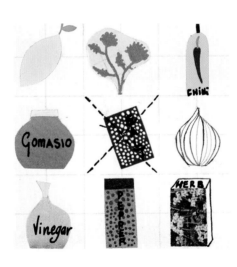

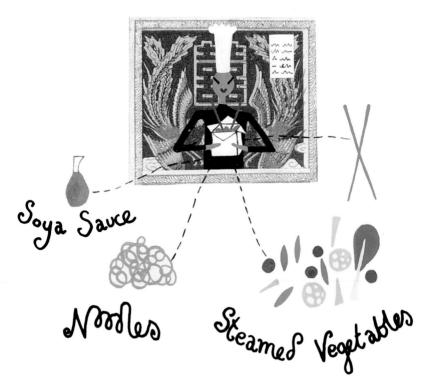

Soya Sauce

Noodles

Steamed Vegetables

86 **Far from being a bad
to go choice, a Chinese meal can
be nutritious and low-fat.**
Get plain noodles or steamed rice
and some steamed vegetables.
Look for favorite flavorings like
garlic, ginger and lemon grass. Oh,
and ask them to hold the
monosodium glutamate. If they
sound unsure they can do so, say
you're allergic to it; that should
get the right reaction.

87 Most coffee bars offer a choice of milk to make your cappuccino frothy. Remember to ask for semi-skimmed or extra skinny if you want to be that way (a cup of whole milk contains 150 calories, a cup of skimmed milk only 85). And don't worry, your mug of milky coffee will still taste the same.

88 Rich sauces are a slimmer's suicide, which is why eating out can be so stressful. When every menu choice includes Hollandaise or Béarnaise sauce (both made from egg yolks and butter—say no more), ask for your sauce on the side. Then you can have one tablespoonful and hand the rest back before you're tempted to eat all of it. As a rule, opt for a red sauce (tomato-based) rather than a white one (butter, milk, cream—all your basic nightmares), and ask if the chef can go easy with the oil. It shouldn't be a problem; if you meet resistance, you can be sure what you're about to eat hasn't been freshly made.

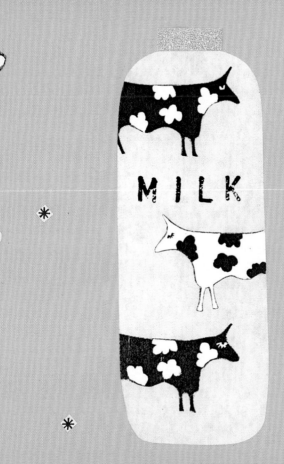

89 **Soup bars are the healthiest fast food in town.** A bowl of soup is nourishing, warming, and easy to digest, and, with literally hundreds of possibilities, soup's also a good way to increase the fluid in your diet. Calorie counters will love soup too, as it's slimming and filling, but make wise choices (vegetable-based soups are best) and hold the croutons, parmesan cheese, and cream toppings.

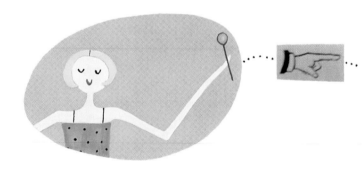

---

90 Everyone overeats once in a while. When you wake up the next day still feeling full of food, have a body-cleansing breakfast of fruit to give your liver something worthwhile to work on.

Lunchtime should be a small plate of oily fish (think mackerel, sardines, or salmon) with salad, which provides healthy fats to help counteract last night's not-so-healthy ones.

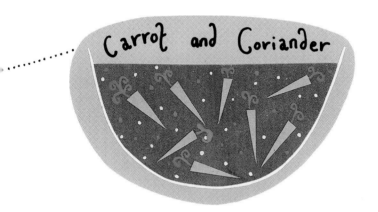

Carrot and Coriander

91 **Choose carefully and a pizza can be far from fattening.** Rule one is to order a thin 'n' crispy pizza, not a big thick wedge of dough. Next, ask for low-fat cheese or look for a cheese-free topping. Then request that the extra room be filled up with fresh vegetables and you've just got yourself the most wholesome pizza in town.

92 **Need a chocolate fix on the run?** You can make chocolate healthier if you buy a brand made from 70 percent cocoa solids. This makes it far less sugar-laden and so rich that a little should go a long way.

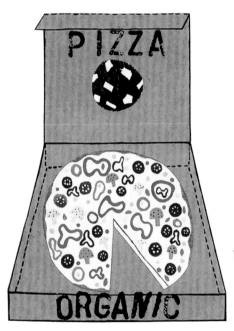

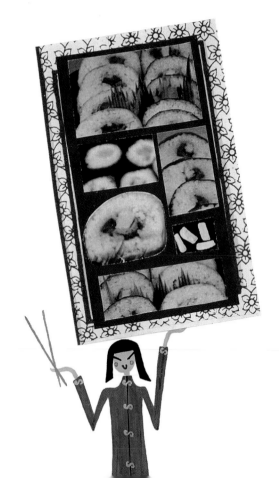

93 **Treat yourself to a Japanese meal and you're sure to feel fabulous the next day.** Seafood or vegetable sushi is low in fat and high in nutrition. Spice it up with slivers of ginger and a sprinkling of soy sauce, and make sure there's a helping of seaweed in there somewhere to boost your healthy brownie points.

94 Eat out at a macrobiotic restaurant and discover the Eastern principles of a yin and yang diet. A yin personality is easy-going, creative, patient, and peaceful, while a yang person is dynamic, alert, assertive, and focused. Followers believe that by eating certain foods you can change the way you behave. For instance, yang foods can make you more confident and able to achieve your goals, while eating too many yin foods can leave you insecure and lethargic. Decide if you need to be more yin or more yang, then make the right choices. Yin foods include eggs, fish, meat, and vegetables that grow downward like carrots and turnips. Yang foods include fruit, vegetables that grow upward, sugar, coffee, and alcohol. Cooking styles can also make food more yin (raw, steaming, and quick-boiling) or yang (frying, baking, and stewing).

95 You can't go wrong with vegetables. Right? Wrong. Some restaurant chefs still think vegetables are boring without drowning them in a butter sauce. Here's what to avoid:

Tempura—you'll just about make out a sliver of vegetable under the deep fried batter.

Fritters—more frying.

Au gratin—vegetables topped with a crispy cheese sauce.

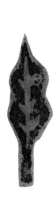
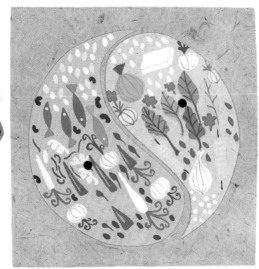
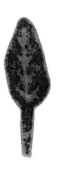

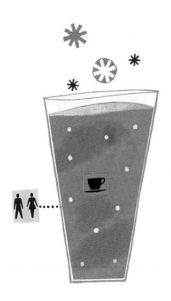

96 No time to eat? Drop into a juice bar and order up a storm to keep your energy levels buzzing. Fresh fruit and vegetables are easy for your body to absorb fast, plus they're filling so you won't go hungry.

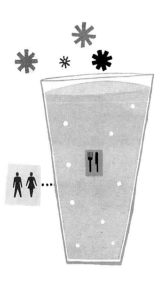

97 **For added nutritional value, ask for a dash of one of these popular extras:**

Wheat germ—contains vitamin E, protein, and iron

Spirulina—contains protein, minerals, and vitamins

Ginseng—works as a caffeine-free stimulant

Brewer's Yeast—contains a bunch of B vitamins.

98 **Can't stay away from your old fast-food haunts?** Then change your choices. A regular burger (i.e. small, no cheese), plus a "garden salad" (no French fries allowed) and a small soda or milk shake (low fat if possible) won't win you any nutrition awards. But it also won't clog up your arteries and pile on the pounds.

99 **Many restaurant waiters bring a basket of bread to your table before you've had a chance to pick up the menu.** By all means take advantage of this (although it'll probably be added to your bill), but don't butter your bread or dunk in olive oil unless you want to clock up about 100 calories a tablespoon. It's true that vegetable oils have less saturated fat and no cholesterol, but they're still dieting disasters. And beware bread that comes ready oiled like Italian foccacia. Don't know your panini from your pumpernickel? Then put it in your paper napkin and see whether it leaves an oily spot.

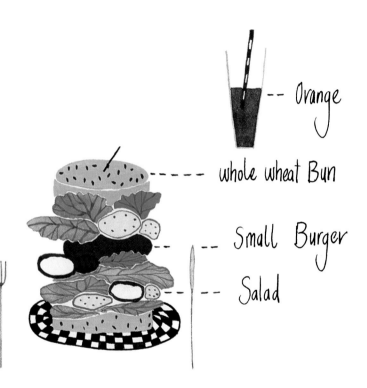

Orange

whole wheat Bun

Small Burger

Salad

100 **When you just kept on eating even when your stomach was begging for mercy,** don't finish your meal with a filling cappuccino or a wide-awake espresso. What you need is a cup of peppermint tea to aid digestion in time for bedtime.

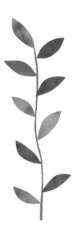

Copyright © MQ Publications Ltd 2002

Text © Liz Wilde 2002
Illustrations © Carol Morley 2002
Interior Design: Philippa Jarvis
Series Editor: Kate John

Time Warner Books are published by
Time Warner Trade Publishing
1271 Ave. of the Americas
New York, NY 10020

Visit our Web site at www.twbookmark.com

 An AOL Time Warner Company

Printed in China
First printing: 10 9 8 7 6 5 4 3 2 1

Library of Congress Control Number: 2001097169

ISBN: 1-931722-08-0